Transform Your Health: A Comprehensive Guide to Diabetes Weight Loss

Unleash the power of a healthy lifestyle and take control of your diabetes with this informative eBook. Discover proven strategies to shed those extra pounds, lower your blood sugar levels, and improve your overall well-being. Each recipe details the carb content to help in controlling your blood sugars.

Table of Contents

Chapter 1: Understanding Diabetes and Weight Loss

The Connection Between Diabetes and Weight

Type 2 diabetes and obesity are closely linked, with about 85% of people with type 2 diabetes being overweight or obese (CDC, 2021). Excess fat, particularly around the abdomen, can contribute to insulin resistance and impaired glucose tolerance, which are hallmarks of type 2 diabetes.

Weight Loss as a Diabetes Management Strategy

Research has consistently shown that losing even a small amount of weight can have significant benefits for diabetes management, including improved blood sugar control, lower HbA1c levels, reduced medication requirements, and decreased risk of diabetes-related complications (Boule et al., 2001; Toilet et al., 2001; Knowler et al., 2002).

Setting Realistic Goals

When embarking on a diabetes weight loss journey, it's essential to set realistic and achievable goals. Aim for a gradual weight loss of 1-2 pounds per week, as this approach is more sustainable and associated with long-term success.

Chapter 2: Importance of a Balanced Diet

Components of a Balanced Diet

A balanced diet for diabetes weight loss includes a variety of nutrient-dense foods from all food groups. These include fruits, vegetables, whole grains, lean proteins, and healthy fats.

Reducing Added Sugars and Refined Carbohydrates

Reducing the consumption of added sugars and refined carbohydrates is crucial for managing blood sugar levels and achieving weight loss. These foods can cause rapid spikes in blood sugar, followed by a quick crash, leading to increased hunger and potential overeating.

Portion Control and Mindful Eating

Implementing portion control and practicing mindful eating can help control calorie intake and prevent overeating. Paying attention to hunger and fullness cues and savouring each bite can contribute to a more enjoyable and sustainable eating experience.

Chapter 3: Macronutrients and Diabetes Weight Loss

Carbohydrates and Diabetes Management

Carbohydrates are the primary source of glucose in the body, and managing carbohydrate intake is essential for maintaining stable blood sugar levels. Focus on consuming complex, fibre-rich carbohydrates, such as whole grains, legumes, fruits, and vegetables, while limiting simple, refined carbohydrates.

The Role of Protein in Diabetes Weight Loss

Protein is important for maintaining muscle mass and satiety during weight loss. Incorporate lean protein sources, such as chicken, fish, tofu, and low-fat dairy, into your meals to support a healthy weight and optimal blood sugar management.

Healthy Fats: Friends, Not Foes

Healthy fats, such as monounsaturated and polyunsaturated fats, can help improve insulin sensitivity and support weight loss. Incorporate sources like avocados, nuts, seeds, and olive oil into your diet to reap the benefits.

Chapter 4: Exercise for Diabetes Management

Aerobic Exercise

Aerobic exercise, such as walking, jogging, cycling, or swimming, can help improve insulin sensitivity, reduce body fat, and lower blood sugar levels. Aim for at least 150 minutes of moderate-intensity aerobic exercise per week.

Resistance Training

Resistance training, such as weightlifting or bodyweight exercises, can help build muscle mass and improve glucose control. Aim for at least two resistance training sessions per week, focusing on all major muscle groups.

Flexibility and Balance Training

Incorporating flexibility and balance exercises, such as yoga or tai chi, can help improve overall fitness, reduce stress, and provide additional benefits for diabetes weight loss.

Chapter 5: Emotional Well-being and Weight Loss

Coping with Emotional Eating

Emotional eating can be a significant barrier to successful weight loss and diabetes management. Identifying triggers, practicing stress reduction techniques, and seeking support from a mental health professional can help address emotional eating and foster a healthier relationship with food.

The Importance of Self-Compassion

Cultivating self-compassion and reframing negative self-talk can help promote a positive mindset and support long-term weight loss success. Be patient, kind, and understanding with yourself as you navigate your diabetes weight loss journey.

Building a Support System

Surrounding yourself with a supportive network of friends, family, and healthcare professionals can enhance your motivation, accountability, and overall well-being during your diabetes weight loss journey.

Chapter 6: Sleep and Diabetes

The Impact of Sleep on Diabetes and Weight

Sleep plays a crucial role in diabetes management and weight loss. Poor sleep quality or insufficient sleep can lead to insulin resistance, increased appetite, and impaired glucose control.

Tips for Optimizing Sleep

Establishing a consistent sleep schedule, creating a relaxing bedtime routine, and ensuring a sleep-conducive environment can help improve sleep quality and duration.

Addressing Sleep Disorders

If you suspect that you may have a sleep disorder, such as sleep pane, consult with your healthcare professional to receive proper diagnosis and treatment.

Chapter 7: Monitoring Progress and Adjusting Your Plan

Tracking Blood Sugar, Weight, and Other Indicators

Regularly monitor blood sugar levels, weight, and other relevant health indicators to track your progress and make necessary adjustments to your diabetes weight loss plan.

Evaluating Your Success

Celebrate non-scale victories, such as improved energy levels and mood, increased strength, and better blood sugar control. Acknowledge that weight loss is not always linear and focus on the overall positive changes in your health.

Adjusting Your Plan as Needed

As you progress through your diabetes weight loss journey, you may need to adjust your diet, exercise, or other lifestyle factors to continue seeing results. Stay open to making changes and seeking support from your healthcare team.

Chapter 8: Recipes for Delicious and Nutritious Meals

CHICKEN

Here are 20 chicken-based dinner ideas for a single person who is a diabetic wishing to lose weight. I have detailed the ingredients, carb counts, and methods for each recipe. Enjoy!

1. Lemon Herb Chicken with Roasted Asparagus

Serves: 1

Ingredients:

* 4 oz boneless and skinless chicken breast (carbs: 0g)

* 1 cup asparagus, trimmed (carbs: 4g)

* 1 teaspoon olive oil (carbs: 0g)

* 1/2 teaspoon lemon juice (carbs: 1g)

* 1/4 teaspoon dried thyme (carbs: 0g)

* 1/4 teaspoon dried rosemary (carbs: 0g)

* Salt and pepper

Method:

1. Preheat the oven to 400°F (200°C).

2. Brush the chicken breast with 1/2 teaspoon olive oil and season

with salt, pepper, thyme, and rosemary.

3. Place the chicken breast on a baking sheet lined with parchment paper.

4. Toss the asparagus with the remaining 1/2 teaspoon olive oil, lemon juice, salt, and pepper.

5. Arrange the asparagus around the chicken breast.

6. Bake for 20-25 minutes or until the chicken is cooked through and the asparagus is tender.

Total Carbs: 5g

2. Chicken and Vegetable Kabobs

Serves: 1

Ingredients:

* 4 oz boneless and skinless chicken breast (carbs: 0g)

* 1/4 cup red bell pepper, cut into 1-inch cubes (carbs: 2g)

* 1/4 cup zucchini, cut into 1-inch cubes (carbs: 1g)

* 1/4 cup red onion, cut into 1-inch cubes (carbs: 2g)

* 1 tablespoon olive oil (carbs: 0g)

* 1/2 teaspoon dried oregano (carbs: 0g)

* 1/2 teaspoon dried basil (carbs: 0g)

* Salt and pepper

Method:

1. Preheat the grill or grill pan to medium-high heat.

2. Cut the chicken breast into 1-inch cubes.

3. In a medium bowl, mix chicken, bell pepper, zucchini, red onion, 1/2 tablespoon olive oil, oregano, basil, salt, and pepper.

4. Thread the chicken and vegetables onto skewers.

5. Brush the skewers with the remaining 1/2 tablespoon olive oil.

6. Grill for 10-12 minutes, turning occasionally, or until the chicken is cooked through.

Total Carbs: 5g

3. Chicken Caesar Salad

Serves: 1

Ingredients:

* 2 oz grilled chicken breast, sliced (carbs: 0g)

* 2 cups romaine lettuce, chopped (carbs: 3g)

* 1 tablespoon Caesar dressing (carbs: 1g)

* 1/4 cup shaved parmesan cheese (carbs: 1g)

* 1/2 teaspoon lemon juice (carbs: 1g)

* Salt and pepper

Method:

1. In a large bowl, mix romaine lettuce, Caesar dressing, lemon juice, salt, and pepper.

2. Add the sliced chicken breast and shaved parmesan cheese.

3. Toss to combine and serve.

Total Carbs: 6g

4. Chicken Fajita Bowl

Serves: 1

Ingredients:

* 4 oz boneless and skinless chicken breast (carbs: 0g)

* 1/4 cup bell pepper, sliced (carbs: 2g)

* 1/4 cup onion, sliced (carbs: 2g)

* 1/4 cup canned black beans, drained and rinsed (carbs: 6g)

* 1/4 cup canned corn, drained and rinsed (carbs: 9g)

* 1/4 cup cooked brown rice (carbs: 22g)

* 1/2 teaspoon olive oil (carbs: 0g)

* 1/4 teaspoon cumin (carbs: 0g)

* 1/4 teaspoon paprika (carbs: 0g)

* 1/4 teaspoon garlic powder (carbs: 0g)

* Salt and pepper

Method:

1. Heat 1/2 teaspoon olive oil in a skillet over medium heat.

2. Cook the chicken breast for 5-7 minutes per side or until cooked through.

3. Remove the chicken from the skillet and set aside.

4. Add bell pepper and onion to the skillet and cook until tender.

5. Slice the cooked chicken breast.

6. In a bowl, mix brown rice, black beans, corn, chicken, and sautéed vegetables.

7. Season with cumin, paprika, garlic powder, salt, and pepper.

Total Carbs: 41g

5. Chicken Teriyaki with Broccoli

Serves: 1

Ingredients:

* 4 oz boneless and skinless chicken breast (carbs: 0g)
* 1 cup broccoli florets (carbs: 10g)
* 1/4 cup teriyaki sauce (carbs: 15g)
* 1 teaspoon sesame oil (carbs: 0g)
* Salt and pepper

Method:

1. Heat sesame oil in a skillet over medium heat.

2. Season the chicken breast with salt and pepper.

3. Cook the chicken breast for 5-7 minutes per side or until cooked through.

4. Remove the chicken from the skillet and set aside.

5. Add the broccoli florets to the skillet and cook until tender.

6. Add the teriyaki sauce to the skillet and stir to combine.

7. Slice the cooked chicken breast and add it to the skillet.

8. Stir to coat the chicken and broccoli in the teriyaki sauce.

Total Carbs: 25g

6. Chicken Shawarma Salad

Serves: 1

Ingredients:

* 4 oz grilled chicken breast, sliced (carbs: 0g)

* 2 cups mixed greens (carbs: 3g)

* 1/4 cup tomato, diced (carbs: 2g)

* 1/4 cup cucumber, diced (carbs: 1g)

* 1/4 cup red onion, thinly sliced (carbs: 2g)

* 1 tablespoon tahini sauce (carbs: 2g)

* 1/2 teaspoon lemon juice (carbs: 1g)

* 1/2 teaspoon dried parsley (carbs: 0g)

* Salt and pepper

Method:

1. In a large bowl, mix mixed greens, tomato, cucumber, and red onion.

2. In a small bowl, whisk tahini sauce, lemon juice, parsley, salt,

and pepper.

3. Pour the tahini dressing over the salad and toss to combine.

4. Add the sliced chicken breast on top of the salad.

Total Carbs: 11g

7. Chicken and Mushroom Stroganoff

Serves: 1

Ingredients:

* 4 oz boneless and skinless chicken breast (carbs: 0g)

* 1/2 cup mushrooms, sliced (carbs: 2g)

* 1/4 cup reduced-fat sour cream (carbs: 4g)

* 1/4 cup canned cream of mushroom soup (carbs: 6g)

* 1 tablespoon whole milk (carbs: 1g)

* 1/4 teaspoon dried thyme (carbs: 0g)

* 1/4 teaspoon dried parsley (carbs: 0g)

* Salt and pepper

Method:

1. Cut the chicken breast into thin strips.

2. Heat a skillet over medium heat and cook the chicken breast for 5-7 minutes or until cooked through.

3. Remove the chicken from the skillet and set aside.

4. In the same skillet, cook the mushrooms until tender.

5. Add the cooked chicken breast back into the skillet.

6. In a small bowl, mix sour cream, cream of mushroom soup, milk, thyme, parsley, salt, and pepper.

7. Pour the sauce over the chicken and mushrooms.

8. Simmer for 5-7 minutes or until heated through.

Total Carbs: 13g

8. Chicken Cordon Bleu

Serves: 1

Ingredients:

* 4 oz boneless and skinless chicken breast (carbs: 0g)

* 1 slice ham (carbs: 1g)

* 1 slice Swiss cheese (carbs: 0g)

* 1/2 tablespoon Dijon mustard (carbs: 1g)

* 1/4 teaspoon garlic powder (carbs: 0g)

* 1/4 teaspoon paprika (carbs: 0g)

* Salt and pepper

Method:

1. Preheat the oven to 350°F (180°C).

2. Cut the chicken breast in half horizontally to create two equal pieces.

3. Place a slice of ham and Swiss cheese on one piece of the chicken

breast.

4. Place the other piece of chicken breast on top to create a sandwich.

5. Secure with toothpicks.

6. In a small bowl, mix Dijon mustard, garlic powder, paprika, salt, and pepper.

7. Brush the mustard mixture over the chicken sandwich.

8. Bake for 25-30 minutes or until the chicken is cooked through.

Total Carbs: 2g

9. Chicken Parmesan

Serves: 1

Ingredients:

* 4 oz boneless and skinless chicken breast (carbs: 0g)

* 1/4 cup marinara sauce (carbs: 6g)

* 1/4 cup shredded mozzarella cheese (carbs: 1g)

* 1/4 cup whole wheat breadcrumbs (carbs: 12g)

* 1/2 tablespoon grated Parmesan cheese (carbs: 1g)

* 1/2 teaspoon dried basil (carbs: 0g)

* 1/2 teaspoon dried oregano (carbs: 0g)

* 1/2 tablespoon olive oil (carbs: 0g)

* Salt and pepper

Method:

1. Preheat the oven to 400°F (200°C).

2. Season the chicken breast with salt and pepper.

3. In a small bowl, mix breadcrumbs, Parmesan cheese, basil, oregano, salt, and pepper.

4. Brush the chicken breast with olive oil and coat it in the breadcrumb mixture.

5. Place the chicken breast on a baking sheet lined with parchment paper.

6. Top the chicken breast with marinara sauce and shredded mozzarella cheese.

7. Bake for 20-25 minutes or until the chicken is cooked through and the cheese is melted.

Total Carbs: 20g

10. Chicken and Vegetable Stir-Fry

Serves: 1

Ingredients:

* 4 oz boneless and skinless chicken breast (carbs: 0g)

* 1/4 cup bell pepper, sliced (carbs: 2g)

* 1/4 cup zucchini, sliced (carbs: 1g)

* 1/4 cup carrot, sliced (carbs: 3g)

* 1/4 cup red onion, sliced (carbs: 2g)

* 1/4 cup canned bamboo shoots, drained (carbs: 2g)

* 1/4 cup canned water chestnuts, drained (carbs: 2g)

* 1 tablespoon reduced-sodium soy sauce (carbs: 2g)

* 1 teaspoon sesame oil (carbs: 0g)

* 1/4 teaspoon dried ginger (carbs: 0g)

* Salt and pepper

Method:

1. Cut the chicken breast into thin strips.

2. Heat sesame oil in a skillet over medium heat.

3. Cook the chicken breast for 5-7 minutes or until cooked through.

4. Remove the chicken from the skillet and set aside.

5. In the same skillet, cook the vegetables until tender.

6. Add the cooked chicken breast and bamboo shoots back into the skillet.

7. Stir in soy sauce and ginger.

8. Simmer for 5-7 minutes or until heated through.

Total Carbs: 14g

11. Chicken and Spinach Salad with Almonds and Feta

Serves: 1

Ingredients:

* 2 oz grilled chicken breast, sliced (carbs: 0g)
* 2 cups baby spinach (carbs: 1g)
* 1/4 cup almonds, sliced (carbs: 3g)
* 1/4 cup feta cheese, crumbled (carbs: 2g)
* 1/4 cup red onion, thinly sliced (carbs: 2g)
* 1 tablespoon olive oil (carbs: 0g)
* 1 tablespoon balsamic vinegar (carbs: 3g)
* 1/2 teaspoon dried oregano (carbs: 0g)
* Salt and pepper

Method:

1. In a large bowl, mix spinach, almonds, feta cheese, and red onion.

2. In a small bowl, whisk olive oil, balsamic vinegar, oregano, salt, and pepper.

3. Pour the dressing over the salad and toss to combine.

4. Add the sliced chicken breast on top of the salad.

Total Carbs: 9g

12. Chicken and Sweet Potato Shepherd's Pie

Serves: 1

Ingredients:

* 4 oz boneless and skinless chicken breast (carbs: 0g)

* 1/2 cup cooked sweet potato, mashed (carbs: 24g)

* 1/4 cup canned peas, drained (carbs: 10g)

* 1/4 cup canned corn, drained (carbs: 9g)

* 1/4 cup canned green beans, drained (carbs: 4g)

* 1/4 cup reduced-fat cheddar cheese, shredded (carbs: 1g)

* 1/4 teaspoon dried thyme (carbs: 0g)

* 1/4 teaspoon dried rosemary (carbs: 0g)

* 1/4 teaspoon garlic powder (carbs: 0g)

* Salt and pepper

Method:

1. Preheat the oven to 400°F (200°C).

2. Cut the chicken breast into small pieces.

3. Heat a skillet over medium heat and cook the chicken breast for 5-7 minutes or until cooked through.

4. Remove the chicken from the skillet and set aside.

5. In the same skillet, cook the peas, corn, and green beans until tender.

6. In a small bowl, mix the cooked chicken and vegetables.

7. Season the mixture with thyme, rosemary, garlic powder, salt, and pepper.

8. Transfer the mixture to a small oven-safe dish.

9. Top with mashed sweet potato and shredded cheddar cheese.

10. Bake for 15-20 minutes or until the cheese is melted and the top is golden brown.

Total Carbs: 49g

13. Chicken and Avocado Salad

Serves: 1

Ingredients:

* 2 oz grilled chicken breast, sliced (carbs: 0g)
* 1 cup mixed greens (carbs: 3g)
* 1/4 cup avocado, diced (carbs: 2g)
* 1/4 cup cherry tomatoes, halved (carbs: 3g)
* 1/4 cup red onion, thinly sliced (carbs: 2g)
* 1 tablespoon olive oil (carbs: 0g)
* 1 tablespoon lemon juice (carbs: 1g)
* 1/2 teaspoon dried parsley (carbs: 0g)
* Salt and pepper

Method:

1. In a large bowl, mix mixed greens, avocado, cherry tomatoes, and red onion.
2. In a small bowl, whisk olive oil, lemon juice, parsley, salt, and pepper.
3. Pour the dressing over the salad and toss to combine.

4. Add the sliced chicken breast on top of the salad.

Total Carbs: 11g

14. Chicken and Broccoli Rabe with Garlic

Serves: 1

Ingredients:

* 4 oz boneless and skinless chicken breast (carbs: 0g)

* 1 cup broccoli rabe, chopped (carbs: 5g)

* 1/4 cup chicken broth (carbs: 1g)

* 1/4 teaspoon dried garlic (carbs: 0g)

* 1/4 teaspoon red pepper flakes (carbs: 0g)

* Salt and pepper

Method:

1. Heat a skillet over medium heat and cook the chicken breast for 5-7 minutes per side or until cooked through.

2. Remove the chicken from the skillet and set aside.

3. In the same skillet, add broccoli rabe, chicken broth, garlic, red pepper flakes, salt, and pepper.

4. Cook until the broccoli rabe is tender.

5. Slice the cooked chicken breast and add it back into the skillet.

6. Stir to combine and simmer for 5-7 minutes or until heated through.

Total Carbs: 6g

15. Chicken and Pineapple Fried Rice

Serves: 1

Ingredients:

* 4 oz boneless and skinless chicken breast (carbs: 0g)
* 1/4 cup canned pineapple, drained and chopped (carbs: 12g)
* 1/4 cup cooked brown rice (carbs: 22g)
* 1/4 cup frozen peas, thawed (carbs: 6g)
* 1/4 cup frozen carrots, thawed (carbs: 5g)
* 1/4 cup scallions, chopped (carbs: 2g)
* 1/4 teaspoon dried garlic (carbs: 0g)
* 1/4 teaspoon dried ginger (carbs: 0g)
* Salt and pepper

Method:

1. Cut the chicken breast into small pieces.

2. Heat a skillet over medium heat and cook the chicken breast for 5-7 minutes or until cooked through.

3. Remove the chicken from the skillet and set aside.

4. In the same skillet, add brown rice, peas, carrots, and scallions.

5. Cook until the vegetables are tender.

6. Add the cooked chicken breast and pineapple back into the

skillet.

7. Stir in garlic and ginger.

8. Simmer for 5-7 minutes or until heated through.

Total Carbs: 47g

16. Chicken and Kale Salad with Lemon Dressing

Serves: 1

Ingredients:

* 2 oz grilled chicken breast, sliced (carbs: 0g)

* 2 cups kale, chopped (carbs: 2g)

* 1/4 cup red onion, thinly sliced (carbs: 2g)

* 1/4 cup red bell pepper, sliced (carbs: 2g)

* 1/4 cup cucumber, sliced (carbs: 1g)

* 1 tablespoon olive oil (carbs: 0g)

* 1 tablespoon lemon juice (carbs: 1g)

* 1/2 teaspoon dried dill (carbs: 0g)

* Salt and pepper

Method:

1. In a large bowl, mix kale, red onion, red bell pepper, and cucumber.

2. In a small bowl, whisk olive oil, lemon juice, dill, salt, and pepper.

3. Pour the dressing over the salad and toss to combine.

4. Add the sliced chicken breast on top of the salad.

Total Carbs: 8g

17. Chicken and Stuffed Bell Peppers

Serves: 1

Ingredients:

* 4 oz boneless and skinless chicken breast (carbs: 0g)
* 1/2 cup cooked brown rice (carbs: 22g)
* 1/4 cup canned black beans, drained and rinsed (carbs: 6g)
* 1/4 cup canned corn, drained (carbs: 9g)
* 1/4 cup canned diced tomatoes (carbs: 5g)
* 1/4 cup cheddar cheese, shredded (carbs: 1g)
* 1/4 teaspoon cumin (carbs: 0g)
* 1/4 teaspoon paprika (carbs: 0g)
* 1/4 teaspoon chili powder (carbs: 0g)
* Salt and pepper
* 1 bell pepper, halved and deseeded

Method:

1. Preheat the oven to 350°F (180°C).

2. Cut the chicken breast into small pieces.

3. Heat a skillet over medium heat and cook the chicken breast for 5-7 minutes or until cooked through.

4. Remove the chicken from the skillet and set aside.

5. In the same skillet, mix brown rice, black beans, corn, diced tomatoes, cheddar cheese, cumin, paprika, chili powder, salt, and pepper.

6. Add the cooked chicken breast to the rice mixture and stir to combine.

7. Spoon the chicken and rice mixture into the bell pepper halves.

8. Place the stuffed bell peppers on a baking sheet lined with parchment paper.

9. Bake for 25-30 minutes or until the bell peppers are tender.

Total Carbs: 43g

18. Chicken and Berry Spinach Salad

Serves: 1

Ingredients:

* 2 oz grilled chicken breast, sliced (carbs: 0g)

* 2 cups baby spinach (carbs: 1g)

* 1/4 cup mixed berries, such as blueberries, raspberries, and strawberries (carbs: 10g)

* 1/4 cup red onion, thinly sliced (carbs: 2g)

* 1/4 cup almonds, sliced (carbs: 3g)

* 1/4 cup crumbled feta cheese (carbs: 2g)

* 1 tablespoon balsamic vinegar (carbs: 3g)

* 1 tablespoon olive oil (carbs: 0g)

* 1/2 teaspoon dried basil (carbs: 0g)

* Salt and pepper

Method:

1. In a large bowl, mix spinach, mixed berries, red onion, almonds, and feta cheese.

2. In a small bowl, whisk balsamic vinegar, olive oil, basil, salt, and pepper.

3. Pour the dressing over the salad and toss to combine.

4. Add the sliced chicken breast on top of the salad.

Total Carbs: 21g

19. Chicken and Vegetable Skewers with Lemon Dill Sauce

Serves: 1

Ingredients:

* 4 oz boneless and skinless chicken breast (carbs: 0g)

* 1/4 cup bell pepper, cut into 1-inch chunks (carbs: 2g)

* 1/4 cup zucchini, cut into 1-inch chunks (carbs: 1g)

* 1/4 cup red onion, cut into 1-inch chunks (carbs: 2g)

* 1/4 cup cherry tomatoes (carbs: 4g)

* 1/4 cup canned artichoke hearts, drained and quartered (carbs: 5g)

* 1/2 cup plain Greek yogurt (carbs: 6g)

* 1/4 teaspoon dried dill (carbs: 0g)

* 1/2 teaspoon lemon zest (carbs: 0g)

* 1/2 teaspoon lemon juice (carbs: 1g)

* Salt and pepper

Method:

1. Preheat the grill or grill pan to medium-high heat.

2. Cut the chicken breast into 1-inch chunks.

3. In a medium bowl, mix chicken, bell pepper, zucchini, red onion, cherry tomatoes, and artichoke hearts.

4. Season the mixture with salt and pepper.

5. Thread the chicken and vegetable chunks onto skewers.

6. Grill the skewers for 10-12 minutes or until the chicken is cooked through.

7. In a small bowl, mix Greek yogurt, dill, lemon zest, lemon juice, salt, and pepper.

8. Serve the chicken and vegetable skewers with the lemon dill sauce.

Total Carbs: 21g

20. Chicken and Mushroom Gravy over Cauliflower Mash

Serves: 1

Ingredients:

* 4 oz boneless and skinless chicken breast (carbs: 0g)
* 1/2 cup mushrooms, sliced (carbs: 2g)
* 1/2 cup chicken broth (carbs: 1g)
* 1/4 cup reduced-fat milk (carbs: 2g)
* 1/4 teaspoon dried thyme (carbs: 0g)
* 1/4 teaspoon dried rosemary (carbs: 0g)
* 1/4 teaspoon garlic powder (carbs: 0g)
* Salt and pepper
* 1 cup cauliflower, cooked and mashed (carbs: 5g)

Method:

1. Preheat the oven to 350°F (180°C).

2. Season the chicken breast with salt and pepper.

3. Heat a skillet over medium heat and cook the chicken breast for 5-7 minutes per side or until cooked through.

4. Remove the chicken from the skillet and set aside.

5. In the same skillet, cook the mushrooms until tender.

6. Add chicken broth, milk, thyme, rosemary, and garlic powder.

7. Bring the mixture to a boil and simmer for 5-7 minutes or until the sauce thickens.

8. Slice the cooked chicken breast and add it back into the skillet.

9. Serve the chicken and mushroom gravy over cauliflower mash.

Total Carbs: 13g

I hope you enjoy these chicken dinner ideas for a single diabetic person wishing to lose weight! Remember to adjust the recipes to your personal preferences and taste. Bon appétit!

FISH

<u>1. Baked Lemon Herb Salmon</u>

Serves: 1

Ingredients:

* 4 oz salmon fillet, skin removed (carbs: 0g)
* 1/2 teaspoon olive oil (carbs: 0g)
* 1 lemon, sliced (carbs: 6g)
* 1/2 teaspoon dried dill (carbs: 0g)
* 1/2 teaspoon dried parsley (carbs: 0g)
* Salt and pepper

Method:

1. Preheat the oven to 400°F (200°C).

2. Place the salmon fillet on a baking sheet lined with parchment paper.

3. Brush the salmon with 1/2 teaspoon olive oil.

4. Top the salmon with lemon slices, dill, parsley, salt, and pepper.

5. Bake for 12-15 minutes or until the salmon is cooked through.

Total Carbs: 6g

2. Mediterranean Grilled Tuna Steak

Serves: 1

Ingredients:

* 4 oz tuna steak (carbs: 0g)
* 1/2 teaspoon olive oil (carbs: 0g)
* 1/2 teaspoon dried oregano (carbs: 0g)
* 1/2 teaspoon dried basil (carbs: 0g)
* 1/2 teaspoon garlic powder (carbs: 0g)
* Salt and pepper
* 1/4 cup cherry tomatoes, halved (carbs: 2g)
* 1/4 cup cucumber, diced (carbs: 1g)
* 1/4 cup red onion, thinly sliced (carbs: 2g)
* 1/4 cup Kalamata olives, pitted and sliced (carbs: 1g)
* 1/4 cup feta cheese, crumbled (carbs: 2g)
* 1 tablespoon red wine vinegar (carbs: 1g)
* 1 tablespoon olive oil (carbs: 0g)

Method:

1. Preheat a grill or grill pan to medium-high heat.

2. Brush the tuna steak with 1/2 teaspoon olive oil and season with oregano, basil, garlic powder, salt, and pepper.

3. Grill the tuna steak for 4-5 minutes per side or until desired doneness.

4. In a medium bowl, mix cherry tomatoes, cucumber, red onion, Kalamata olives, feta cheese, red wine vinegar, and 1 tablespoon olive oil.

5. Serve the grilled tuna steak with the Mediterranean salad.

Total Carbs: 9g

<u>3. Spicy Baked Cod</u>

Serves: 1

Ingredients:

* 4 oz cod fillet (carbs: 0g)
* 1/2 teaspoon olive oil (carbs: 0g)
* 1/2 teaspoon chili powder (carbs: 0g)
* 1/4 teaspoon paprika (carbs: 0g)
* 1/4 teaspoon garlic powder (carbs: 0g)
* 1/4 teaspoon cumin (carbs: 0g)
* Salt and pepper
* 1/4 cup bell pepper, diced (carbs: 2g)
* 1/4 cup red onion, diced (carbs: 2g)
* 1/4 cup tomato, diced (carbs: 2g)
* 1/4 cup canned black beans, drained and rinsed (carbs: 6g)
* 1/4 cup corn, drained and rinsed (carbs: 9g)
* 1/4 cup cilantro, chopped (carbs: 0g)

* 1/4 avocado, diced (carbs: 2g)

* 1 tablespoon lime juice (carbs: 2g)

* 1/2 jalapeno, seeds removed and finely chopped (carbs: 0g)

Method:

1. Preheat the oven to 400°F (200°C).

2. Mix chili powder, paprika, garlic powder, cumin, salt, and pepper in a small bowl.

3. Brush the cod fillet with 1/2 teaspoon olive oil and coat it with the spice mixture.

4. Place the cod fillet on a baking sheet lined with parchment paper.

5. Bake for 12-15 minutes or until the cod flakes easily with a fork.

6. In a medium bowl, mix bell pepper, red onion, tomato, black beans, corn, cilantro, avocado, lime juice, and jalapeno.

7. Serve the spicy baked cod with the black bean and corn salsa.

Total Carbs: 27g

4. Lemon Butter Tilapia

Serves: 1

Ingredients:

* 4 oz tilapia fillet (carbs: 0g)

* 1/2 teaspoon olive oil (carbs: 0g)

* 1/4 cup unsalted butter (carbs: 0g)

* 1 lemon, juiced and zested (carbs: 6g)

* 1 clove garlic, minced (carbs: 1g)

* 1/4 teaspoon dried thyme (carbs: 0g)

* Salt and pepper

* 1/4 cup asparagus, trimmed (carbs: 2g)

* 1/4 cup green beans, trimmed (carbs: 2g)

Method:

1. Preheat a skillet over medium heat and add 1/2 teaspoon olive oil.

2. Season the tilapia fillet with salt and pepper.

3. Cook the tilapia fillet for 3-4 minutes per side or until cooked through.

4. In a small saucepan, melt the butter over low heat.

5. Add lemon juice, lemon zest, garlic, and thyme, stirring frequently.

6. Cook the asparagus and green beans in a separate skillet for 5-7 minutes or until tender.

7. Serve the tilapia drizzled with the lemon butter sauce and the cooked asparagus and green beans on the side.

Total Carbs: 11g

5. Garlic Herb Trout

Serves: 1

Ingredients:

* 4 oz trout fillet (carbs: 0g)

* 1/2 teaspoon olive oil (carbs: 0g)

* 1 clove garlic, minced (carbs: 1g)

* 1/2 teaspoon dried thyme (carbs: 0g)

* 1/2 teaspoon dried rosemary (carbs: 0g)

* 1/2 teaspoon dried parsley (carbs: 0g)

* Salt and pepper

* 1/4 cup cherry tomatoes, halved (carbs: 2g)

* 1/4 cup cucumber, diced (carbs: 1g)

* 1/4 cup red onion, thinly sliced (carbs: 2g)

* 1/4 cup Kalamata olives, pitted and sliced (carbs: 1g)

* 1/4 cup feta cheese, crumbled (carbs: 2g)

* 1 tablespoon lemon juice (carbs: 2g)

* 1 tablespoon olive oil (carbs: 0g)

Method:

1. Preheat the oven to 400°F (200°C).

2. Mix garlic, thyme, rosemary, parsley, salt, and pepper in a small bowl.

3. Brush the trout fillet with 1/2 teaspoon olive oil and coat it with the herb mixture.

4. Place the trout fillet on a baking sheet lined with parchment paper.

5. Bake for 12-15 minutes or until the trout is cooked through.

6. In a medium bowl, mix cherry tomatoes, cucumber, red onion, Kalamata olives, feta cheese, lemon juice, and 1 tablespoon olive oil.

7. Serve the garlic herb trout with the Mediterranean salad.

Total Carbs: 11g

6. Grilled Shrimp with Mango Salsa

Serves: 1

Ingredients:

* 6 oz shrimp, peeled and deveined (carbs: 0g)

* 1/2 teaspoon olive oil (carbs: 0g)

* 1/2 teaspoon dried oregano (carbs: 0g)

* 1/2 teaspoon garlic powder (carbs: 0g)

* Salt and pepper

* 1/4 cup mango, diced (carbs: 15g)

* 1/4 cup black beans, drained and rinsed (carbs: 6g)

* 1/4 cup red bell pepper, diced (carbs: 2g)

* 1/4 cup red onion, diced (carbs: 2g)

* 1/4 cup cilantro, chopped (carbs: 0g)

* 1/2 jalapeno, seeds removed and finely chopped (carbs: 0g)

* 1 tablespoon lime juice (carbs: 2g)

Method:

1. Preheat a grill or grill pan to medium-high heat.

2. Toss the shrimp with 1/2 teaspoon olive oil, oregano, garlic powder, salt, and pepper.

3. Grill the shrimp for 2-3 minutes per side or until pink and cooked through.

4. In a medium bowl, mix mango, black beans, red bell pepper, red onion, cilantro, jalapeno, and lime juice.

5. Serve the grilled shrimp with the mango salsa.

Total Carbs: 27g

7. Lemon Parmesan Baked Cod

Serves: 1

Ingredients:

* 4 oz cod fillet (carbs: 0g)

* 1/2 teaspoon olive oil (carbs: 0g)

* 1 lemon, juiced and zested (carbs: 6g)

* 1/4 cup grated Parmesan cheese (carbs: 2g)

* 1/4 teaspoon dried basil (carbs: 0g)

* 1/4 teaspoon dried oregano (carbs: 0g)

* Salt and pepper

Method:

1. Preheat the oven to 400°F (200°C).

2. Mix lemon juice, lemon zest, Parmesan cheese, basil, oregano, salt, and pepper in a small bowl.

3. Brush the cod fillet with 1/2 teaspoon olive oil.

4. Coat the cod fillet with the Parmesan mixture.

5. Place the cod fillet on a baking sheet lined with parchment paper.

6. Bake for 12-15 minutes or until the cod flakes easily with a fork.

Total Carbs: 8g

8. Seared Tuna with Avocado Salad

Serves: 1

Ingredients:

* 4 oz tuna steak (carbs: 0g)

* 1/2 teaspoon olive oil (carbs: 0g)

* Salt and pepper

* 1/2 avocado, diced (carbs: 4g)

* 1/2 cup cucumber, diced (carbs: 2g)

* 1/2 cup cherry tomatoes, halved (carbs: 2g)

* 1/4 cup red onion, thinly sliced (carbs: 2g)

* 1/4 cup cilantro, chopped (carbs: 0g)

* 1 tablespoon lime juice (carbs: 2g)

* 1 tablespoon olive oil (carbs: 0g)

Method:

1. Preheat a skillet over medium-high heat and add 1/2 teaspoon olive oil.

2. Season the tuna steak with salt and pepper.

3. Sear the tuna steak for 1-2 minutes per side or until desired doneness.

4. In a medium bowl, mix avocado, cucumber, cherry tomatoes, red onion, cilantro, lime juice, and 1 tablespoon olive oil.

5. Serve the seared tuna steak with the avocado salad.

Total Carbs: 10g

9. Grilled Halibut with Lemon Garlic Butter

Serves: 1

Ingredients:

* 4 oz halibut fillet (carbs: 0g)

* 1/2 teaspoon olive oil (carbs: 0g)

* Salt and pepper

* 1/4 cup unsalted butter (carbs: 0g)

* 1 lemon, juiced and zested (carbs: 6g)

* 1 clove garlic, minced (carbs: 1g)

* 1/4 teaspoon dried thyme (carbs: 0g)

Method:

1. Preheat a grill or grill pan to medium-high heat.

2. Brush the halibut fillet with 1/2 teaspoon olive oil and season with salt and pepper.

3. Grill the halibut fillet for 4-5 minutes per side or until cooked through.

4. In a small saucepan, melt the butter over low heat.

5. Add lemon juice, lemon zest, garlic, thyme, salt, and pepper, stirring frequently.

6. Serve the grilled halibut with the lemon garlic butter.

Total Carbs: 7g

10. Herb Crusted Salmon

Serves: 1

Ingredients:

* 4 oz salmon fillet, skin removed (carbs: 0g)

* 1/2 teaspoon olive oil (carbs: 0g)

* 1/4 cup panko breadcrumbs (carbs: 16g)

* 1/4 cup grated Parmesan cheese (carbs: 2g)

* 1/4 teaspoon dried thyme (carbs: 0g)

* 1/4 teaspoon dried rosemary (carbs: 0g)

* 1/4 teaspoon dried parsley (carbs: 0g)

* Salt and pepper

* 1/4 cup lemon slices (carbs: 2g)

Method:

1. Preheat the oven to 400°F (200°C).

2. Mix panko breadcrumbs, Parmesan cheese, thyme, rosemary, parsley, salt, and pepper in a small bowl.

3. Brush the salmon fillet with 1/2 teaspoon olive oil.

4. Coat the salmon fillet with the breadcrumb mixture.

5. Place the salmon fillet on a baking sheet lined with parchment paper.

6. Top the salmon with lemon slices.

7. Bake for 12-15 minutes or until the salmon is cooked through.

Total Carbs: 20g

11. Baked Flounder with Tomato and Herbs

Serves: 1

Ingredients:

* 4 oz flounder fillet (carbs: 0g)

* 1/2 teaspoon olive oil (carbs: 0g)

* 1/2 cup cherry tomatoes, halved (carbs: 2g)

* 1/4 cup red onion, thinly sliced (carbs: 2g)

* 1/4 cup Kalamata olives, pitted and sliced (carbs: 1g)

* 1/4 cup cilantro, chopped (carbs: 0g)

* 1/2 lemon, sliced (carbs: 3g)

* 1/4 cup white wine (carbs: 3g)

* 1/4 teaspoon dried basil (carbs: 0g)

* 1/4 teaspoon dried thyme (carbs: 0g)

* Salt and pepper

Method:

1. Preheat the oven to 400°F (200°C).

2. Mix cherry tomatoes, red onion, Kalamata olives, cilantro, salt, and pepper in a small bowl.

3. Place the flounder fillet on a baking sheet lined with parchment paper.

4. Top the flounder fillet with the tomato mixture and lemon slices.

5. Pour the white wine over the fish.

6. Sprinkle basil and thyme over the fish.

7. Bake for 12-15 minutes or until the flounder is cooked through.

Total Carbs: 11g

12. Pan-Seared Scallops with Spinach and Bacon

Serves: 1

Ingredients:

* 6 oz scallops (carbs: 0g)

* 1/2 teaspoon olive oil (carbs: 0g)

* Salt and pepper

* 2 slices bacon, cooked and crumbled (carbs: 0g)

* 1/4 cup red onion, thinly sliced (carbs: 2g)

* 2 cups fresh spinach (carbs: 1g)

* 1/2 lemon, juiced (carbs: 2g)

Method:

1. Preheat a skillet over medium-high heat and add 1/2 teaspoon olive oil.

2. Season the scallops with salt and pepper.

3. Sear the scallops for 2-3 minutes per side or until caramelized.

4. In the same skillet, cook the red onion until tender.

5. Add spinach and cook until wilted.

6. Add crumbled bacon and lemon juice.

7. Serve the scallops with the spinach and bacon mixture.

Total Carbs: 5g

13. Lemon Dill Baked Tilapia

Serves: 1

Ingredients:

* 4 oz tilapia fillet (carbs: 0g)

* 1/2 teaspoon olive oil (carbs: 0g)

* 1/4 cup lemon slices (carbs: 2g)

* 1/4 cup vegetable broth (carbs: 1g)

* 1/4 teaspoon dried dill (carbs: 0g)

* 1/4 teaspoon dried parsley (carbs: 0g)

* Salt and pepper

Method:

1. Preheat the oven to 350°F (180°C).

2. Place the tilapia fillet on a baking sheet lined with parchment paper.

3. Top the tilapia fillet with lemon slices.

4. Pour the vegetable broth over the fish.

5. Sprinkle dill and parsley over the fish.

6. Bake for 12-15 minutes or until the tilapia flakes easily with a fork.

Total Carbs: 3g

14. Pesto Crusted Salmon

Serves: 1

Ingredients:

* 4 oz salmon fillet, skin removed (carbs: 0g)

* 1/2 teaspoon olive oil (carbs: 0g)

* 1/4 cup pesto sauce (carbs: 2g)

* 1/4 cup panko breadcrumbs (carbs: 16g)

* 1/4 teaspoon garlic powder (carbs: 0g)

* Salt and pepper

Method:

1. Preheat the oven to 400°F (200°C).

2. Mix pesto sauce, panko breadcrumbs, garlic powder, salt, and pepper in a small bowl.

3. Brush the salmon fillet with 1/2 teaspoon olive oil.

4. Coat the salmon fillet with the pesto mixture.

5. Place the salmon fillet on a baking sheet lined with parchment paper.

6. Bake for 12-15 minutes or until the salmon is cooked through.

Total Carbs: 18g

15. Grilled Swordfish with Spicy Rub

Serves: 1

Ingredients:

* 4 oz swordfish steak (carbs: 0g)

* 1/2 teaspoon olive oil (carbs: 0g)

* 1/2 teaspoon chili powder (carbs: 0g)

* 1/4 teaspoon paprika (carbs: 0g)

* 1/4 teaspoon garlic powder (carbs: 0g)

* 1/4 teaspoon cumin (carbs: 0g)

* Salt and pepper

* 1/4 cup cherry tomatoes, halved (carbs: 2g)

* 1/4 cup red onion, thinly sliced (carbs: 2g)

* 1/4 cup cilantro, chopped (carbs: 0g)

* 1/2 jalapeno, seeds removed and finely chopped (carbs: 0g)

* 1 tablespoon lime juice (carbs: 2g)

Method:

1. Preheat a grill or grill pan to medium-high heat.

2. Mix chili powder, paprika, garlic powder, cumin, salt, and pepper in a small bowl.

3. Brush the swordfish steak with 1/2 teaspoon olive oil.

4. Coat the swordfish steak with the spice mixture.

5. Grill the swordfish steak for 4-5 minutes per side or until cooked through.

6. In a medium bowl, mix cherry tomatoes, red onion, cilantro, jalapeno, and lime juice.

7. Serve the grilled swordfish steak with the salsa.

Total Carbs: 8g

16. Lemon Butter Poached Tilapia

Serves: 1

Ingredients:

* 4 oz tilapia fillet (carbs: 0g)

* 1/2 cup low-sodium chicken broth (carbs: 1g)

* 1/4 cup unsalted butter (carbs: 0g)

* 1 lemon, juiced and zested (carbs: 6g)

* 1 clove garlic, minced (carbs: 1g)

* 1/4 teaspoon dried thyme (carbs: 0g)

* Salt and pepper

Method:

1. In a skillet, bring chicken broth to a simmer.

2. Add butter, lemon juice, lemon zest, garlic, thyme, salt, and pepper.

3. Stir until butter has melted.

4. Add tilapia fillet and simmer for 5-7 minutes or until cooked through.

Total Carbs: 8g

17. Spicy Blackened Tuna

Serves: 1

Ingredients:

* 4 oz tuna steak (carbs: 0g)

* 1/2 teaspoon olive oil (carbs: 0g)

* 1/2 teaspoon chili powder (carbs: 0g)

* 1/4 teaspoon paprika (carbs: 0g)

* 1/4 teaspoon garlic powder (carbs: 0g)

* 1/4 teaspoon cayenne pepper (carbs: 0g)

* 1/4 teaspoon dried oregano (carbs: 0g)

* Salt and pepper

Method:

1. Preheat a skillet over medium-high heat and add 1/2 teaspoon olive oil.

2. Mix chili powder, paprika, garlic powder, cayenne pepper, oregano, salt, and pepper in a small bowl.

3. Coat the tuna steak with the spice mixture.

4. Sear the tuna steak for 1-2 minutes per side or until desired doneness.

Total Carbs: 0g

<u>18. Herb and Lemon Baked Cod</u>

Serves: 1

Ingredients:

* 4 oz cod fillet (carbs: 0g)

* 1/2 teaspoon olive oil (carbs: 0g)

* 1/4 cup lemon slices (carbs: 2g)

* 1/4 cup vegetable broth (carbs: 1g)

* 1/4 teaspoon dried basil (carbs: 0g)

* 1/4 teaspoon dried thyme (carbs: 0g)

* 1/4 teaspoon garlic powder (carbs: 0g)

* Salt and pepper

Method:

1. Preheat the oven to 350°F (180°C).

2. Place the cod fillet on a baking sheet lined with parchment paper.

3. Top the cod fillet with lemon slices.

4. Pour the vegetable broth over the fish.

5. Sprinkle basil, thyme, and garlic powder over the fish.

6. Bake for 12-15 minutes or until the cod flakes easily with a fork.

Total Carbs: 3g

19. Blackened Catfish with Avocado Salsa

Serves: 1

Ingredients:

* 4 oz catfish fillet (carbs: 0g)

* 1/2 teaspoon olive oil (carbs: 0g)

* 1/2 teaspoon chili powder (carbs: 0g)

* 1/4 teaspoon paprika (carbs: 0g)

* 1/4 teaspoon garlic powder (carbs: 0g)

* 1/4 teaspoon dried oregano (carbs: 0g)

* 1/4 teaspoon onion powder (carbs: 0g)

* Salt and pepper

* 1/4 cup avocado, diced (carbs: 4g)

* 1/4 cup red onion, diced (carbs: 2g)

* 1/4 cup red bell pepper, diced (carbs: 2g)

* 1/4 cup cilantro, chopped (carbs: 0g)

* 1/2 lime, juiced (carbs: 2g)

Method:

1. Preheat a skillet over medium-high heat and add 1/2 teaspoon olive oil.

2. Mix chili powder, paprika, garlic powder, dried oregano, onion powder, salt, and pepper in a small bowl.

3. Coat the catfish fillet with the spice mixture.

4. Sear the catfish fillet for 4-5 minutes per side or until cooked through.

5. In a medium bowl, mix avocado, red onion, red bell pepper, cilantro, and lime juice.

6. Serve the blackened catfish with the avocado salsa.

Total Carbs: 10g

20. Grilled Sesame Tuna Steak

Serves: 1

Ingredients:

* 4 oz tuna steak (carbs: 0g)
* 1/2 teaspoon sesame oil (carbs: 0g)
* 1/4 cup soy sauce (carbs: 2g)
* 1/4 teaspoon ginger, grated (carbs: 0g)
* 1/4 teaspoon garlic, minced (carbs: 0g)
* 1 tablespoon sesame seeds (carbs: 2g)
* Salt and pepper

Method:

1. Preheat a grill or grill pan to medium-high heat.

2. Mix sesame oil, soy sauce, ginger, and garlic in a small bowl.

3. Marinate the tuna steak in the soy sauce mixture for 10 minutes.

4. Coat the tuna steak with sesame seeds.

5. Grill the tuna steak for 1-2 minutes per side or until desired doneness.

Total Carbs: 4g

I hope you enjoy these healthy, low-carb fish recipes for a single person! Remember to adjust the recipes to your personal preferences and taste. Bon appétit!

LAMB

Here are 10 lamb recipes for 1 serving for a person who is diabetic and wishes to lose weight, detailing the amount of carbs per ingredient and the total carbs at the end.

Recipe 1: Lamb and Tomato Salad

Ingredients and Carb Counts

* 3 oz (85g) lamb loin, grilled and sliced (0g carbohydrates)

* 2 cups mixed greens (1g carbohydrates)

* 1 medium tomato, diced (2g carbohydrates)

* 1/4 medium cucumber, diced (0.5g carbohydrates)

* 1 tbsp crumbled feta cheese (0g carbohydrates)

* 1 tbsp olive oil (0g carbohydrates)

* 1 tbsp balsamic vinegar (0g carbohydrates)

Method

1. Grill the lamb loin to desired doneness and let it rest for a few minutes before slicing.

2. In a large bowl, combine the mixed greens, diced tomato, and diced cucumber.

3. Top the salad with the sliced lamb and crumbled feta cheese.

4. Drizzle the olive oil and balsamic vinegar over the salad.

5. Toss the salad gently to combine and serve.

Total Carbohydrates

3.5g carbohydrates (tomato, cucumber, mixed greens)

Recipe 2: Lamb and Avocado Wrap

Ingredients and Carb Counts

* 2 oz (57g) lamb loin, grilled and sliced (0g carbohydrates)

* 1 medium whole grain or low-carb tortilla (15g carbohydrates)

* 1/2 medium avocado, sliced (3.5g carbohydrates)

* 1/4 cup shredded lettuce (0.5g carbohydrates)

* 1 medium tomato, sliced (1g carbohydrates)

* 1 tbsp hummus (0g carbohydrates)

Method

1. Grill the lamb loin to desired doneness and let it rest for a few minutes before slicing.

2. Lay the tortilla flat on a plate.

3. Spread the hummus evenly over the tortilla.

4. Arrange the sliced lamb, avocado, lettuce, and tomato on the tortilla.

5. Roll the tortilla tightly and slice it in half diagonally.

Total Carbohydrates

19g carbohydrates (tortilla, avocado, tomato, lettuce)

Recipe 3: Lamb Skewers with Tzatziki Sauce

Ingredients and Carb Counts

* 2 oz (57g) lamb loin, cut into 1-inch pieces (0g carbohydrates)

* 1/2 medium zucchini, sliced into rounds (1g carbohydrates)

* 1/2 medium bell pepper, cut into 1-inch pieces (1g carbohydrates)

* 1 tbsp olive oil (0g carbohydrates)

* 1/4 cup tzatziki sauce (1g carbohydrates)

Method

1. Preheat a grill or grill pan over medium heat.

2. Thread the lamb, zucchini, and bell pepper slices onto a skewer.

3. Brush the skewers with olive oil.

4. Grill the skewers for 5-6 minutes, turning them frequently to cook evenly.

5. Serve the skewers with tzatziki sauce on the side.

Total Carbohydrates

3g carbohydrates (zucchini, bell pepper, tzatziki sauce)

Recipe 4: Lamb and Mushroom Stir-Fry

Ingredients and Carb Counts

* 3 oz (85g) lamb loin, sliced (0g carbohydrates)

* 1 cup mixed vegetables (2g carbohydrates)

* 1 tbsp olive oil (0g carbohydrates)

* 1 clove garlic, minced (0g carbohydrates)

* 1 tbsp low-sodium soy sauce (0g carbohydrates)

* 1 tbsp water (0g carbohydrates)

Method

1. Heat the olive oil in a large skillet over medium heat.

2. Add the sliced lamb and cook for 3-4 minutes, until browned.

3. Add the mixed vegetables and garlic to the skillet. Continue cooking for 3-4 minutes, until the vegetables are tender.

4. Stir in the low-sodium soy sauce and water.

5. Cook for an additional minute, allowing the Flavors to meld.

6. Serve and enjoy.

Total Carbohydrates

2g carbohydrates (mixed vegetables)

Recipe 5: Lamb and Asparagus Salad

Ingredients and Carb Counts

* 3 oz (85g) lamb loin, grilled and sliced (0g carbohydrates)

* 1 cup asparagus, blanched and chopped (2g carbohydrates)

* 1 cup mixed greens (1g carbohydrates)

* 1 tbsp vinaigrette dressing (0g carbohydrates)

Method

1. Grill the lamb loin to desired doneness and let it rest for a few minutes before slicing.

2. Blanch the asparagus by boiling it for 3-4 minutes, then plunging it into ice water to stop the cooking process.

3. Chop the asparagus into bite-sized pieces.

4. In a large bowl, combine the mixed greens and chopped asparagus.

5. Add the sliced lamb to the bowl.

6. Drizzle the vinaigrette dressing over the salad and toss to combine.

Total Carbohydrates

3g carbohydrates (asparagus, mixed greens)

Recipe 6: Lamb and Cauliflower Fried Rice

Ingredients and Carb Counts

* 3 oz (85g) lamb loin, diced (0g carbohydrates)

* 1 cup cauliflower rice (3g carbohydrates)

* 1/2 cup frozen peas and carrots (4g carbohydrates)

* 1 tbsp soy sauce (0g carbohydrates)

* 1 tbsp vegetable oil (0g carbohydrates)

* 1 clove garlic, minced (0g carbohydrates)

* 1 egg, beaten (0g carbohydrates)

Method

1. Heat the vegetable oil in a large skillet over medium heat.

2. Add the diced lamb and cook for 3-4 minutes, until browned.

3. Add the cauliflower rice, frozen peas and carrots, and minced garlic to the skillet. Cook for 5-6 minutes, until the cauliflower rice is tender.

4. Stir in the soy sauce.

5. Push the lamb and vegetables to one side of the skillet and pour the beaten egg onto the other side. Scramble the egg and stir it into the lamb and vegetable mixture.

Total Carbohydrates

7g carbohydrates (cauliflower rice, frozen peas and carrots)

Recipe 7: Lamb and Spinach Soup

Ingredients and Carb Counts

* 3 oz (85g) lamb stew meat, diced (0g carbohydrates)

* 1 cup low-sodium chicken broth (0g carbohydrates)

* 1 cup fresh spinach leaves (1g carbohydrates)

* 1/4 cup chopped onion (1g carbohydrates)

* 1 clove garlic, minced (0g carbohydrates)

* 1 tbsp chopped parsley (0g carbohydrates)

Method

1. Place the diced lamb stew meat, chicken broth, chopped onion, and minced garlic in a pot.

2. Bring the pot to a boil over high heat, then reduce the heat to low and simmer the soup for 30-40 minutes, until the lamb is tender.

3. Stir in the spinach leaves and chopped parsley.

4. Cook for an additional 2-3 minutes, allowing the spinach to wilt.

5. Serve and enjoy.

Total Carbohydrates

2g carbohydrates (spinach, onion)

Recipe 8: Lamb and Roasted Vegetable Bowl

Ingredients and Carb Counts

* 3 oz (85g) lamb loin, diced (0g carbohydrates)
* 1 cup mixed vegetables (2g carbohydrates)
* 1 tbsp olive oil (0g carbohydrates)

Method

1. Preheat the oven to 400°F (200°C).
2. Toss the mixed vegetables in the olive oil and spread them out

on a baking sheet.

3. Roast the vegetables in the preheated oven for 20-25 minutes, until tender and lightly browned.

4. While the vegetables are roasting, cook the diced lamb in a skillet over medium heat for 5-6 minutes, until cooked through.

5. Place the roasted vegetables and cooked lamb in a bowl and serve.

Total Carbohydrates

2g carbohydrates (mixed vegetables)

Recipe 9: Lamb and Green Bean Casserole

Ingredients and Carb Counts

* 3 oz (85g) lamb loin, diced (0g carbohydrates)

* 1 cup green beans, trimmed (3g carbohydrates)

* 1/4 cup canned cream of mushroom soup (2g carbohydrates)

* 1/4 cup canned French fried onions (2g carbohydrates)

* 1 tbsp vegetable oil (0g carbohydrates)

Method

1. Preheat the oven to 375°F (190°C).

2. Heat the vegetable oil in a skillet over medium heat and cook the diced lamb for 5-6 minutes, until cooked through.

3. Steam the green beans until tender.

4. In a casserole dish, combine the cooked lamb, steamed green

beans, and cream of mushroom soup.

5. Bake the casserole for 15-20 minutes, until heated through.

6. Top the casserole with the French-fried onions and bake for an additional 5 minutes.

Total Carbohydrates

7g carbohydrates (green beans, cream of mushroom soup, French fried onions)

Recipe 10: Lamb and Sweet Potato Shepherd's Pie

Ingredients and Carb Counts

* 3 oz (85g) lamb stew meat, diced (0g carbohydrates)
* 1/2 cup mashed sweet potato (10g carbohydrates)
* 1/4 cup frozen peas (2g carbohydrates)
* 1/4 cup frozen carrots (2g carbohydrates)
* 1/4 cup canned corn (2g carbohydrates)
* 1/4 cup canned green beans (0g carbohydrates)
* 1/4 cup canned kidney beans (2g carbohydrates)
* 1/4 cup canned diced tomatoes (1g carbohydrates)
* 1 tbsp tomato paste (0g carbohydrates)
* 1 tsp Worcestershire sauce (0g carbohydrates)
* 1 tbsp vegetable oil (0g carbohydrates)

Method

1. Preheat the oven to 375°F (190°C).

2. Heat the vegetable oil in a skillet over medium heat and cook the diced lamb for 5-6 minutes, until cooked through.

3. In a separate pan, cook the frozen peas, carrots, corn, green beans, and kidney beans until tender.

4. Add the canned diced tomatoes, tomato paste, and Worcestershire sauce to the pan and cook for an additional 2-3 minutes.

5. Spoon the vegetable and lamb mixture into a small casserole dish.

6. Top the mixture with mashed sweet potato.

7. Bake the shepherd's pie for 20-25 minutes, until heated through and the sweet potato is slightly golden.

Total Carbohydrates

21g carbohydrates (mashed sweet potato, frozen peas, frozen carrots, canned corn, canned green beans, canned kidney beans, canned diced tomatoes)

These recipes can be adjusted and modified based on your individual meal plan, preferences, and carbohydrate allowance. Remember to track the carbohydrates in each ingredient and the total carbohydrates in the final dish to ensure you stay within your desired carb range. Enjoy experimenting with these lamb recipes and discovering new favourites!

BEEF

<u>Recipe 1: Beef and Broccoli Stir-Fry</u>

Ingredients and Carb Counts

* 3 oz (85g) beef tenderloin, sliced (0g carbohydrates)

* 1 cup broccoli florets (3g carbohydrates)

* 1 tbsp olive oil (0g carbohydrates)

* 1 tbsp low-sodium soy sauce (0g carbohydrates)

* 1 tbsp water (0g carbohydrates)

* 1 clove garlic, minced (0g carbohydrates)

* 1/2 small onion, sliced (1.5g carbohydrates)

* 1/4 medium bell pepper, sliced (0.5g carbohydrates)

Method

1. Heat the olive oil in a large skillet over medium heat.

2. Add the sliced beef and cook for 3-4 minutes, until browned.

3. Add the broccoli, sliced onion, sliced bell pepper, minced garlic, low-sodium soy sauce, and water.

4. Cook for an additional 5-7 minutes, until the beef is cooked to desired doneness and the broccoli is tender.

5. Serve and enjoy.

Total Carbohydrates

5g carbohydrates (broccoli, onion, bell pepper)

Recipe 2: Beef and Avocado Salad

Ingredients and Carb Counts

* 3 oz (85g) beef tenderloin, grilled and sliced (0g carbohydrates)

* 2 cups mixed greens (2g carbohydrates)

* 1/2 medium avocado, diced (3.5g carbohydrates)

* 1/4 medium bell pepper, sliced (0.5g carbohydrates)

* 1/4 medium cucumber, sliced (0.5g carbohydrates)

* 1 tbsp olive oil (0g carbohydrates)

* 1 tbsp lime juice (0g carbohydrates)

Method

1. Grill the beef tenderloin to desired doneness, then let it rest for a few minutes before slicing.

2. In a large bowl, combine the mixed greens, diced avocado, sliced bell pepper, and sliced cucumber.

3. Top the salad with the sliced beef.

4. In a small bowl, whisk together the olive oil and lime juice.

5. Drizzle the dressing over the salad.

6. Toss the salad gently to combine and serve.

Total Carbohydrates

6.5g carbohydrates (mixed greens, avocado, bell pepper, cucumber)

Recipe 3: Beef and Mushroom Lettuce Wraps

Ingredients and Carb Counts

* 3 oz (85g) beef tenderloin, cooked and diced (0g carbohydrates)
* 1 large lettuce leaf (0g carbohydrates)
* 1/2 cup sliced mushrooms (1g carbohydrates)
* 1 tbsp olive oil (0g carbohydrates)
* 1 tbsp hoisin sauce (1g carbohydrates)
* 1 tsp soy sauce (0g carbohydrates)
* 1/2 tsp grated ginger (0g carbohydrates)

Method

1. Heat the olive oil in a skillet over medium heat.

2. Add the sliced mushrooms and cook for 4-5 minutes, until tender.

3. Add the cooked diced beef, hoisin sauce, soy sauce, and grated ginger to the skillet.

4. Cook for an additional 2-3 minutes, allowing the Flavors to meld.

5. Place the beef and mushroom mixture in the lettuce leaf and serve.

Total Carbohydrates

2g carbohydrates (mushrooms, hoisin sauce)

Recipe 4: Beef and Green Bean Casserole

Ingredients and Carb Counts

* 3 oz (85g) beef tenderloin, diced (0g carbohydrates)

* 1 cup green beans, trimmed (3g carbohydrates)

* 1/4 cup canned cream of mushroom soup (2g carbohydrates)

* 1/4 cup canned French fried onions (2g carbohydrates)

* 1 tbsp vegetable oil (0g carbohydrates)

Method

1. Preheat the oven to 375°F (190°C).

2. Heat the vegetable oil in a skillet over medium heat and cook the diced beef for 5-6 minutes, until cooked through.

3. Steam the green beans until tender.

4. In a casserole dish, combine the cooked beef, steamed green beans, and cream of mushroom soup.

5. Bake the casserole for 15-20 minutes, until heated through.

6. Top the casserole with the French-fried onions and bake for an additional 5 minutes.

Total Carbohydrates

7g carbohydrates (green beans, cream of mushroom soup, French fried onions)

Recipe 5: Beef and Spinach Soup

Ingredients and Carb Counts

* 3 oz (85g) beef tenderloin, diced (0g carbohydrates)
* 1/2 medium onion, chopped (1.5g carbohydrates)
* 1 cup fresh spinach leaves, chopped (0.5g carbohydrates)
* 1 clove garlic, minced (0g carbohydrates)
* 3 cups low-sodium beef broth (0g carbohydrates)
* 1/4 cup canned diced tomatoes (1g carbohydrates)
* 1 tbsp tomato paste (0g carbohydrates)
* 1 tbsp vegetable oil (0g carbohydrates)

Method

1. Heat the vegetable oil in a large pot over medium heat.
2. Add the chopped onion and minced garlic, and cook for 3-4 minutes, until tender.
3. Add the diced beef and cook for an additional 4-5 minutes, until browned.
4. Stir in the chopped spinach leaves, low-sodium beef broth, canned diced tomatoes, and tomato paste.
5. Bring the pot to a boil over high heat, then reduce the heat to low and simmer the soup for 30-40 minutes, until the beef is tender.
6. Serve and enjoy.

Total Carbohydrates

3g carbohydrates (onion, spinach, diced tomatoes)

Recipe 6: Beef and Tomato Sauce over Spaghetti Squash

Ingredients and Carb Counts

* 3 oz (85g) beef tenderloin, diced (0g carbohydrates)

* 1/2 cup canned diced tomatoes (1g carbohydrates)

* 1/2 cup canned tomato sauce (2g carbohydrates)

* 1/2 small onion, chopped (1.5g carbohydrates)

* 1 clove garlic, minced (0g carbohydrates)

* 1 tsp dried basil (0g carbohydrates)

* 1 tsp dried oregano (0g carbohydrates)

* 1/2 medium spaghetti squash (7g carbohydrates)

* 1 tbsp vegetable oil (0g carbohydrates)

Method

1. Preheat the oven to 375°F (190°C).

2. Cut the spaghetti squash in half, scoop out the seeds, and brush the cut sides with vegetable oil.

3. Place the spaghetti squash halves on a baking sheet, cut side down, and bake for 30-40 minutes, until tender.

4. While the spaghetti squash is baking, heat the vegetable oil in a skillet over medium heat.

5. Add the chopped onion, minced garlic, and diced beef. Cook for

5-6 minutes, until the beef is browned.

6. Stir in the canned diced tomatoes, canned tomato sauce, dried basil, and dried oregano.

7. Cook the sauce for 10-15 minutes, allowing the Flavors to meld.

8. Scrape out the spaghetti squash strands from the cooked halves.

9. Serve the beef and tomato sauce over the spaghetti squash.

Total Carbohydrates

11g carbohydrates (spaghetti squash, canned diced tomatoes, canned tomato sauce)

Recipe 7: Beef and Cauliflower Fried Rice

Ingredients and Carb Counts

* 3 oz (85g) beef tenderloin, diced (0g carbohydrates)

* 1 cup cauliflower rice (3g carbohydrates)

* 1/2 small onion, chopped (1.5g carbohydrates)

* 1/2 medium carrot, chopped (2g carbohydrates)

* 2 tbsp frozen peas (1g carbohydrates)

* 2 tbsp canned diced water chestnuts (1g carbohydrates)

* 1 tbsp soy sauce (0g carbohydrates)

* 1/2 tbsp sesame oil (0g carbohydrates)

* 1/2 tbsp olive oil (0g carbohydrates)

Method

1. Heat 1/2 tbsp of olive oil in a skillet over medium heat.

2. Add the diced beef and cook for 5-6 minutes, until browned. Transfer the beef to a plate.

3. In the same skillet, heat the sesame oil.

4. Add the chopped onion and chopped carrot, and cook for 3-4 minutes, until tender.

5. Stir in the cauliflower rice, frozen peas, and canned diced water chestnuts. Cook for an additional 5-7 minutes, until the cauliflower rice is tender.

6. Add the cooked beef, soy sauce, and any accumulated beef juices back to the skillet.

7. Cook for an additional 1-2 minutes, allowing the Flavors to meld.

8. Serve and enjoy.

Total Carbohydrates

8g carbohydrates (cauliflower rice, onion, carrot, peas, water chestnuts)

Recipe 8: Beef and Roasted Vegetable Bowl

Ingredients and Carb Counts

* 3 oz (85g) beef tenderloin, diced (0g carbohydrates)

* 1 cup mixed vegetables (2g carbohydrates)

* 1 tbsp olive oil (0g carbohydrates)

Method

1. Preheat the oven to 400°F (200°C).

2. Toss the mixed vegetables in the olive oil and spread them out on a baking sheet.

3. Roast the vegetables in the preheated oven for 20-25 minutes, until tender and lightly browned.

4. While the vegetables are roasting, cook the diced beef in a skillet over medium heat for 5-6 minutes, until cooked through.

5. Place the roasted vegetables and cooked beef in a bowl and serve.

Total Carbohydrates

2g carbohydrates (mixed vegetables)

Recipe 9: Beef and Mushroom Gravy

Ingredients and Carb Counts

* 3 oz (85g) beef tenderloin, diced (0g carbohydrates)

* 1/2 cup sliced mushrooms (1g carbohydrates)

* 1/2 cup low-sodium beef broth (0g carbohydrates)

* 1/2 tbsp butter (0g carbohydrates)

* 1/2 tbsp all-purpose flour (3g carbohydrates)

* 1/2 tsp dried thyme (0g carbohydrates)

* 1/2 tsp dried rosemary (0g carbohydrates)

Method

1. Heat the butter in a skillet over medium heat.

2. Add the sliced mushrooms and cook for 4-5 minutes, until

tender.

3. Add the diced beef and cook for an additional 4-5 minutes, until browned.

4. Sprinkle the all-purpose flour over the beef and mushrooms. Cook for 1-2 minutes, allowing the flour to absorb the fat.

5. Gradually stir in the low-sodium beef broth, dried thyme, and dried rosemary.

6. Cook the gravy for 5-7 minutes, until thickened.

7. Serve and enjoy.

Total Carbohydrates

4g carbohydrates (mushrooms, all-purpose flour)

Recipe 10: Beef and Sweet Potato Shepherd's Pie

Ingredients and Carb Counts

* 3 oz (85g) beef stew meat, diced (0g carbohydrates)

* 1/2 cup mashed sweet potato (10g carbohydrates)

* 1/4 cup frozen peas (2g carbohydrates)

* 1/4 cup frozen carrots (2g carbohydrates)

* 1/4 cup canned corn (2g carbohydrates)

* 1/4 cup canned green beans (0g carbohydrates)

* 1/4 cup canned diced tomatoes (1g carbohydrates)

* 1 tbsp tomato paste (0g carbohydrates)

* 1 tsp Worcestershire sauce (0g carbohydrates)

* 1 tbsp vegetable oil (0g carbohydrates)

Method

1. Preheat the oven to 375°F (190°C).

2. Heat the vegetable oil in a skillet over medium heat and cook the diced beef for 5-6 minutes, until cooked through.

3. In a separate pan, cook the frozen peas, carrots, corn, green beans, and diced tomatoes until tender.

4. Add the canned diced tomatoes, tomato paste, and Worcestershire sauce to the pan and cook for an additional 2-3 minutes.

5. Spoon the vegetable and lamb mixture into a small casserole dish.

6. Top the mixture with mashed sweet potato.

7. Bake the shepherd's pie for 20-25 minutes, until heated through and the sweet potato is slightly golden.

Total Carbohydrates

21g carbohydrates (mashed sweet potato, frozen peas, frozen carrots, canned corn, canned green beans, canned diced tomatoes)

These recipes can be adjusted and modified based on your individual meal plan, preferences, and carbohydrate allowance. Remember to track the carbohydrates in each ingredient and the total carbohydrates in the final dish to ensure you stay within your desired carb range. Enjoy experimenting with these beef recipes and discovering new favourites!

VEGETARIAN

<u>Recipe 1: Vegetarian Black Bean and Quinoa Bowl</u>

Ingredients and Carb Counts

* 1/4 cup cooked quinoa (12g carbohydrates)

* 1/4 cup cooked black beans (9g carbohydrates)

* 1/2 cup sliced bell peppers (1g carbohydrates)

* 1/2 cup chopped zucchini (1g carbohydrates)

* 1/4 cup canned diced tomatoes (1g carbohydrates)

* 1/2 cup chopped spinach (0g carbohydrates)

* 1/2 tbsp olive oil (0g carbohydrates)

* 1/2 tsp cumin (0g carbohydrates)

* 1/2 tsp chili powder (0g carbohydrates)

* 1/2 tsp garlic powder (0g carbohydrates)

* 1/2 tsp onion powder (0g carbohydrates)

* 1/4 tsp paprika (0g carbohydrates)

* Salt and pepper to taste (0g carbohydrates)

Method

1. Heat the olive oil in a skillet over medium heat.

2. Add the sliced bell peppers and chopped zucchini to the skillet

and cook for 4-5 minutes, until tender.

3. Add the cumin, chili powder, garlic powder, onion powder, and paprika to the skillet.

4. Stir to combine and cook for an additional 1-2 minutes, allowing the spices to toast.

5. Add the cooked quinoa, black beans, canned diced tomatoes, and chopped spinach to the skillet.

6. Mix well and cook for an additional 2-3 minutes, until heated through.

7. Season with salt and pepper to taste.

8. Serve the black bean and quinoa bowl and enjoy.

Total Carbohydrates

26g carbohydrates (quinoa, black beans, bell peppers, zucchini, canned diced tomatoes, spinach)

Recipe 2: Vegetarian Lentil and Vegetable Stir-Fry

Ingredients and Carb Counts

* 1/4 cup cooked lentils (6g carbohydrates)

* 1/2 cup sliced mushrooms (1g carbohydrates)

* 1/2 cup sliced bell peppers (1g carbohydrates)

* 1/2 cup chopped zucchini (1g carbohydrates)

* 1/4 cup canned diced tomatoes (1g carbohydrates)

* 1/2 cup chopped spinach (0g carbohydrates)

* 1/2 tbsp olive oil (0g carbohydrates)

* 1/2 tsp cumin (0g carbohydrates)

* 1/2 tsp coriander (0g carbohydrates)

* 1/2 tsp turmeric (0g carbohydrates)

* 1/2 tsp garlic powder (0g carbohydrates)

* Salt and pepper to taste (0g carbohydrates)

Method

1. Heat the olive oil in a skillet over medium heat.

2. Add the sliced mushrooms, sliced bell peppers, and chopped zucchini to the skillet.

3. Cook for 4-5 minutes, until tender.

4. Add the cumin, coriander, turmeric, and garlic powder to the skillet.

5. Stir to combine and cook for an additional 1-2 minutes, allowing the spices to toast.

6. Add the cooked lentils, canned diced tomatoes, and chopped spinach to the skillet.

7. Mix well and cook for an additional 2-3 minutes, until heated through.

8. Season with salt and pepper to taste.

9. Serve the lentil and vegetable stir-fry and enjoy.

Total Carbohydrates

12g carbohydrates (lentils, mushrooms, bell peppers, zucchini, canned diced tomatoes, spinach)

Recipe 3: Vegetarian Tofu and Broccoli Stir-Fry

Ingredients and Carb Counts

* 3 oz extra-firm tofu, cubed (0g carbohydrates)

* 1/2 cup chopped broccoli florets (1g carbohydrates)

* 1/2 cup sliced bell peppers (1g carbohydrates)

* 1/2 cup chopped zucchini (1g carbohydrates)

* 1/4 cup canned diced tomatoes (1g carbohydrates)

* 1/2 tbsp olive oil (0g carbohydrates)

* 1/2 tsp garlic powder (0g carbohydrates)

* 1/2 tsp onion powder (0g carbohydrates)

* 1/2 tsp ginger (0g carbohydrates)

* 1 tsp soy sauce (0g carbohydrates)

* Salt and pepper to taste (0g carbohydrates)

Method

1. Heat the olive oil in a skillet over medium heat.

2. Add the cubed tofu to the skillet and cook for 4-5 minutes, until golden brown on all sides.

3. Transfer the tofu to a plate and set aside.

4. Add the chopped broccoli, sliced bell peppers, and chopped zucchini to the skillet.

5. Cook for 4-5 minutes, until tender.

6. Add the canned diced tomatoes, garlic powder, onion powder, and ginger to the skillet.

7. Stir to combine and cook for an additional 1-2 minutes, allowing the spices to toast.

8. Add the tofu, soy sauce, and salt and pepper to taste.

9. Mix well and cook for an additional 2-3 minutes, until heated through.

10. Serve the tofu and broccoli stir-fry and enjoy.

Total Carbohydrates

6g carbohydrates (broccoli, bell peppers, zucchini, canned diced tomatoes)

Recipe 4: Vegetarian Chickpea and Spinach Salad

Ingredients and Carb Counts

* 1/4 cup cooked chickpeas (6g carbohydrates)

* 1/2 cup chopped spinach (0g carbohydrates)

* 1/4 cup sliced bell peppers (0.5g carbohydrates)

* 1/4 cup sliced cucumber (0.5g carbohydrates)

* 1/4 cup canned diced tomatoes (0.5g carbohydrates)

* 1 tbsp olive oil (0g carbohydrates)

* 1 tbsp lemon juice (0g carbohydrates)

* 1/2 clove garlic, minced (0g carbohydrates)

* 1/2 tsp dried oregano (0g carbohydrates)

* Salt and pepper to taste (0g carbohydrates)

Method

1. In a bowl, combine the cooked chickpeas, chopped spinach, sliced bell peppers, sliced cucumber, and canned diced tomatoes.

2. In a separate bowl, whisk together the olive oil, lemon juice,

minced garlic, and dried oregano.

3. Drizzle the dressing over the salad and toss gently to combine.

4. Season with salt and pepper to taste.

5. Serve the chickpea and spinach salad and enjoy.

Total Carbohydrates

8g carbohydrates (chickpeas, bell peppers, cucumber, canned diced tomatoes)

Recipe 5: Vegetarian Stuffed Bell Peppers

Ingredients and Carb Counts

* 1/2 medium bell pepper (1g carbohydrates)

* 1/4 cup cooked quinoa (4g carbohydrates)

* 1/4 cup canned black beans (1.5g carbohydrates)

* 1/4 cup canned diced tomatoes (0.5g carbohydrates)

* 1/4 cup chopped zucchini (0.5g carbohydrates)

* 1/2 tbsp olive oil (0g carbohydrates)

* 1/2 tsp cumin (0g carbohydrates)

* 1/2 tsp chili powder (0g carbohydrates)

* 1/2 tsp garlic powder (0g carbohydrates)

* 1/2 tsp onion powder (0g carbohydrates)

* Salt and pepper to taste (0g carbohydrates)

Method

1. Preheat the oven to 375°F (190°C).

2. Cut off the top of the bell pepper and remove the seeds and membranes.

3. Heat the olive oil in a skillet over medium heat.

4. Add the chopped zucchini to the skillet and cook for 2-3 minutes, until tender.

5. Add the cooked quinoa, canned black beans, canned diced tomatoes, and spices to the skillet.

6. Mix well and cook for an additional 2-3 minutes, until heated through.

7. Season with salt and pepper to taste.

8. Stuff the bell pepper with the quinoa and vegetable mixture.

9. Bake the stuffed bell pepper for 20-25 minutes, until the bell pepper is tender.

10. Serve the stuffed bell pepper and enjoy.

Total Carbohydrates

7g carbohydrates (bell pepper, quinoa, black beans, zucchini, canned diced tomatoes)

Recipe 6: Vegetarian Avocado and Cucumber Salad

Ingredients and Carb Counts

* 1/2 medium avocado (3g carbohydrates)

* 1/2 medium cucumber (1g carbohydrates)

* 1/2 cup chopped tomatoes (2g carbohydrates)

* 1/2 tbsp olive oil (0g carbohydrates)

* 1 tbsp lime juice (0g carbohydrates)

* 1/2 tsp dried cilantro (0g carbohydrates)

* Salt and pepper to taste (0g carbohydrates)

Method

1. Cut the avocado and cucumber into bite-sized pieces.

2. In a bowl, combine the avocado, cucumber, and chopped tomatoes.

3. In a separate bowl, whisk together the olive oil, lime juice, and dried cilantro.

4. Drizzle the dressing over the salad and toss gently to combine.

5. Season with salt and pepper to taste.

6. Serve the avocado and cucumber salad and enjoy.

Total Carbohydrates

7g carbohydrates (avocado, cucumber, tomatoes)

Recipe 7: Vegetarian Spaghetti Squash with Marinara Sauce

Ingredients and Carb Counts

* 1 cup cooked spaghetti squash (10g carbohydrates)

* 1/4 cup marinara sauce (3g carbohydrates)

* 1/4 cup chopped onion (1g carbohydrates)

* 1/2 tbsp olive oil (0g carbohydrates)

* 1/2 tsp garlic powder (0g carbohydrates)

* 1/2 tsp dried basil (0g carbohydrates)

* Salt and pepper to taste (0g carbohydrates)

Method

1. Preheat the oven to 400°F (205°C).

2. Cut the spaghetti squash in half lengthwise and scoop out the seeds.

3. Place the spaghetti squash halves on a baking sheet and bake for 30-40 minutes, until tender.

4. Heat the olive oil in a skillet over medium heat.

5. Add the chopped onion to the skillet and cook for 3-4 minutes, until tender.

6. Add the marinara sauce, garlic powder, and dried basil to the skillet.

7. Stir to combine and cook for an additional 2-3 minutes, until heated through.

8. Use a fork to scrape out the spaghetti squash strands.

9. Mix the spaghetti squash strands with the marinara sauce mixture.

10. Season with salt and pepper to taste.

11. Serve the spaghetti squash with marinara sauce and enjoy.

Total Carbohydrates

15g carbohydrates (spaghetti squash, marinara sauce, onion)

Recipe 8: Vegetarian Roasted Vegetables with Tahini Sauce

Ingredients and Carb Counts

* 1 cup chopped vegetables (carrots, broccoli, cauliflower, etc.) (4g carbohydrates)
* 1 tbsp olive oil (0g carbohydrates)
* 1/2 tsp cumin (0g carbohydrates)
* 1/2 tsp coriander (0g carbohydrates)
* Salt and pepper to taste (0g carbohydrates)

Tahini Sauce

* 1 tbsp tahini (2g carbohydrates)
* 1 tbsp lemon juice (0g carbohydrates)
* 1 tbsp water (0g carbohydrates)
* 1/2 clove garlic, minced (0g carbohydrates)
* Salt and pepper to taste (0g carbohydrates)

Method

1. Preheat the oven to 425°F (220°C).

2. Toss the chopped vegetables with olive oil, cumin, coriander, salt, and pepper.

3. Spread the vegetables on a baking sheet and roast for 20-25 minutes, until tender.

4. In a bowl, whisk together the tahini, lemon juice, water, minced garlic, salt, and pepper.

5. Drizzle the tahini sauce over the roasted vegetables.

6. Serve the roasted vegetables with tahini sauce and enjoy.

Total Carbohydrates

10g carbohydrates (vegetables, tahini)

Recipe 9: Vegetarian Mediterranean Quinoa Bowl

Ingredients and Carb Counts

* 1/4 cup cooked quinoa (6g carbohydrates)

* 1/4 cup chopped cucumber (0.5g carbohydrates)

* 1/4 cup chopped tomatoes (1g carbohydrates)

* 1/4 cup chopped red onion (1g carbohydrates)

* 1/4 cup canned chickpeas (3g carbohydrates)

* 1/4 cup crumbled feta cheese (0.5g carbohydrates)

Dressing

* 1 tbsp olive oil (0g carbohydrates)

* 1 tbsp lemon juice (0g carbohydrates)

* 1/2 tsp dried oregano (0g carbohydrates)

* Salt and pepper to taste (0g carbohydrates)

Method

1. In a bowl, combine the cooked quinoa, chopped cucumber, chopped tomatoes, chopped red onion, canned chickpeas, and crumbled feta cheese.

2. In a separate bowl, whisk together the olive oil, lemon juice,

dried oregano, salt, and pepper.

3. Drizzle the dressing over the quinoa bowl and toss gently to combine.

4. Serve the Mediterranean quinoa bowl and enjoy.

Total Carbohydrates

12g carbohydrates (quinoa, cucumber, tomatoes, red onion, chickpeas, feta cheese)

Recipe 10: Vegetarian Egg and Spinach Scramble

Ingredients and Carb Counts

* 1 large egg (0.5g carbohydrates)

* 1/2 cup chopped spinach (0g carbohydrates)

* 1/4 cup chopped bell peppers (0.5g carbohydrates)

* 1/4 cup chopped tomatoes (1g carbohydrates)

* 1 tsp olive oil (0g carbohydrates)

* 1/2 tsp garlic powder (0g carbohydrates)

* 1/2 tsp onion powder (0g carbohydrates)

* Salt and pepper to taste (0g carbohydrates)

Method

1. Heat the olive oil in a skillet over medium heat.

2. Add the chopped bell peppers and chopped tomatoes to the skillet and cook for 2-3 minutes, until tender.

3. Add the chopped spinach, garlic powder, and onion powder to

the skillet.

4. Stir to combine and cook for an additional 1-2 minutes, until the spinach is wilted.

5. Crack the egg into the skillet and scramble with the vegetables.

6. Cook for 2-3 minutes, until the egg is cooked to desired doneness.

7. Season with salt and pepper to taste.

8. Serve the egg and spinach scramble and enjoy.

Total Carbohydrates

2g carbohydrates (bell peppers, tomatoes, spinach)

These vegetarian recipes can be adjusted and modified based on your individual preferences, dietary needs, and carbohydrate allowance. Remember to track the carbohydrates in each ingredient and the total carbohydrates in the final dish to ensure you stay within your desired carb range. Enjoy experimenting with these vegetarian recipes and discovering new favourites!

VEGAN

Recipe 1: Vegan Quinoa and Black Bean Salad

Ingredients and Carb Counts

* 1/4 cup cooked quinoa (12g carbohydrates)

* 1/4 cup cooked black beans (9g carbohydrates)

* 1/2 cup chopped cucumber (0.5g carbohydrates)

* 1/2 cup chopped bell peppers (1g carbohydrates)

* 1/4 cup canned diced tomatoes (1g carbohydrates)

* 1/2 tbsp olive oil (0g carbohydrates)

* 1 tbsp lime juice (0g carbohydrates)

* 1/2 tsp chili powder (0g carbohydrates)

* 1/2 tsp cumin (0g carbohydrates)

* Salt and pepper to taste (0g carbohydrates)

Method

1. In a bowl, combine the cooked quinoa, cooked black beans, chopped cucumber, chopped bell peppers, and canned diced tomatoes.

2. In a separate bowl, whisk together the olive oil, lime juice, chili powder, and cumin.

3. Drizzle the dressing over the quinoa and vegetable mixture.

4. Toss gently to combine.

5. Season with salt and pepper to taste.

6. Serve the quinoa and black bean salad and enjoy.

Total Carbohydrates

24g carbohydrates (quinoa, black beans, cucumber, bell peppers, tomatoes, olive oil, lime juice)

Recipe 2: Vegan Lentil Soup

Ingredients and Carb Counts

* 1/4 cup cooked green lentils (6g carbohydrates)

* 1/2 cup vegetable broth (0g carbohydrates)

* 1/4 cup chopped onion (1.5g carbohydrates)

* 1/4 cup chopped carrots (3g carbohydrates)

* 1/4 cup chopped celery (0.5g carbohydrates)

* 1/2 tsp dried thyme (0g carbohydrates)

* 1/2 tsp dried basil (0g carbohydrates)

* Salt and pepper to taste (0g carbohydrates)

Method

1. In a small saucepan, combine the cooked lentils, vegetable broth, chopped onion, chopped carrots, and chopped celery.

2. Bring the mixture to a simmer over medium heat.

3. Add the dried thyme and dried basil.

4. Cook for 10-15 minutes, until the vegetables are tender.

5. Season with salt and pepper to taste.

6. Serve the lentil soup and enjoy.

Total Carbohydrates

11g carbohydrates (lentils, onion, carrots, celery, thyme, basil)

Recipe 3: Vegan Roasted Vegetables

Ingredients and Carb Counts

* 1 cup chopped vegetables (carrots, bell peppers, zucchini, etc.) (7g carbohydrates)
* 1/2 tbsp olive oil (0g carbohydrates)
* Salt and pepper to taste (0g carbohydrates)

Method

1. Preheat the oven to 425°F (220°C).

2. Toss the chopped vegetables with olive oil, salt, and pepper.

3. Spread the vegetables on a baking sheet and roast for 20-25 minutes, until tender.

4. Serve the roasted vegetables and enjoy.

Total Carbohydrates

7g carbohydrates (vegetables, olive oil)

Recipe 4: Vegan Greek Salad

Ingredients and Carb Counts

* 1 cup chopped cucumber (0.5g carbohydrates)

* 1/2 cup chopped tomatoes (1g carbohydrates)

* 1/4 cup chopped red onion (1g carbohydrates)

* 1/4 cup sliced black olives (0.5g carbohydrates)

* 1 tbsp olive oil (0g carbohydrates)

* 1 tbsp lemon juice (0g carbohydrates)

* 1/2 tsp dried oregano (0g carbohydrates)

* Salt and pepper to taste (0g carbohydrates)

Method

1. In a bowl, combine the chopped cucumber, chopped tomatoes, chopped red onion, and sliced black olives.

2. In a separate bowl, whisk together the olive oil, lemon juice, dried oregano, salt, and pepper.

3. Drizzle the dressing over the Greek salad.

4. Toss gently to combine.

5. Serve the Greek salad and enjoy.

Total Carbohydrates

3g carbohydrates (cucumber, tomatoes, red onion, black olives, olive oil, lemon juice)

Recipe 5: Vegan Chickpea Salad

Ingredients and Carb Counts

* 1/2 cup cooked chickpeas (14g carbohydrates)
* 1/4 cup chopped cucumber (0.5g carbohydrates)
* 1/4 cup chopped bell peppers (1g carbohydrates)
* 1/4 cup chopped red onion (1g carbohydrates)
* 1 tbsp hummus (2g carbohydrates)
* 1/2 tbsp lemon juice (0g carbohydrates)
* 1/2 tsp dried dill (0g carbohydrates)
* Salt and pepper to taste (0g carbohydrates)

Method

1. In a bowl, combine the cooked chickpeas, chopped cucumber, chopped bell peppers, and chopped red onion.

2. In a separate bowl, whisk together the hummus, lemon juice, dried dill, salt, and pepper.

3. Drizzle the dressing over the chickpea salad.

4. Toss gently to combine.

5. Serve the chickpea salad and enjoy.

Total Carbohydrates

20g carbohydrates (chickpeas, cucumber, bell peppers, red onion, hummus)

Recipe 6: Vegan Stuffed Bell Peppers

Ingredients and Carb Counts

* 1/2 cup cooked quinoa (12g carbohydrates)

* 1/2 cup cooked black beans (9g carbohydrates)

* 1/4 cup canned diced tomatoes (1g carbohydrates)

* 1/4 cup chopped onion (1.5g carbohydrates)

* 1/4 cup chopped bell peppers (1g carbohydrates)

* 1/2 tbsp olive oil (0g carbohydrates)

* 1/2 tsp cumin (0g carbohydrates)

* 1/2 tsp chili powder (0g carbohydrates)

* Salt and pepper to taste (0g carbohydrates)

Method

1. Preheat the oven to 375°F (190°C).

2. In a bowl, combine the cooked quinoa, cooked black beans, canned diced tomatoes, chopped onion, and chopped bell peppers.

3. In a skillet, heat the olive oil over medium heat.

4. Add the cumin and chili powder.

5. Cook for 1 minute, until fragrant.

6. Add the quinoa and black bean mixture to the skillet.

7. Cook for 5 minutes, until heated through.

8. Season with salt and pepper to taste.

9. Stuff the mixture into a halved bell pepper.

10. Place the stuffed bell pepper on a baking sheet and bake for 20-25 minutes, until tender.

11. Serve the stuffed bell pepper and enjoy.

Total Carbohydrates

26g carbohydrates (quinoa, black beans, diced tomatoes, onion, bell peppers, olive oil, cumin, chili powder)

Recipe 7: Vegan Tofu Stir-Fry

Ingredients and Carb Counts

* 3 oz firm tofu (0g carbohydrates)
* 1/2 cup chopped vegetables (broccoli, bell peppers, carrots, etc.) (7g carbohydrates)
* 1 tbsp soy sauce (0g carbohydrates)
* 1/2 tbsp rice vinegar (0g carbohydrates)
* 1 tsp sesame oil (0g carbohydrates)
* 1 tsp garlic powder (0g carbohydrates)
* 1 tsp ginger (0g carbohydrates)
* Salt and pepper to taste (0g carbohydrates)

Method

1. Prepare the tofu by pressing it to remove excess water.
2. Cut the tofu into cubes.
3. In a skillet, heat the sesame oil over medium heat.
4. Add the garlic powder and ginger.
5. Cook for 1 minute, until fragrant.
6. Add the tofu to the skillet.
7. Cook for 5 minutes, until browned on all sides.

8. Add the chopped vegetables to the skillet.

9. Cook for 5 minutes, until tender.

10. In a separate bowl, whisk together the soy sauce and rice vinegar.

11. Pour the soy sauce and rice vinegar mixture over the tofu and vegetable mixture.

12. Cook for 2 minutes, until heated through.

13. Season with salt and pepper to taste.

14. Serve the tofu stir-fry and enjoy.

Total Carbohydrates

7g carbohydrates (vegetables, soy sauce, rice vinegar)

Recipe 8: Vegan Spaghetti Squash with Marinara Sauce

Ingredients and Carb Counts

* 1 cup cooked spaghetti squash (8g carbohydrates)
* 1/2 cup marinara sauce (6g carbohydrates)
* 1/4 cup chopped onion (1.5g carbohydrates)
* 1/2 tbsp olive oil (0g carbohydrates)
* Salt and pepper to taste (0g carbohydrates)

Method

1. Preheat the oven to 400°F (200°C).

2. Cut the spaghetti squash in half and scoop out the seeds.

3. Place the spaghetti squash on a baking sheet and bake for 40-50

minutes, until tender.

4. In a skillet, heat the olive oil over medium heat.

5. Add the chopped onion and cook for 5 minutes, until tender.

6. Add the marinara sauce to the skillet.

7. Cook for 10 minutes, until heated through.

8. Scrape the spaghetti squash out of the shell with a fork.

9. Serve the spaghetti squash with marinara sauce and enjoy.

Total Carbohydrates

15g carbohydrates (spaghetti squash, marinara sauce, onion)

Recipe 9: Vegan Roasted Chickpeas

Ingredients and Carb Counts

* 1/2 cup cooked chickpeas (14g carbohydrates)
* 1/2 tbsp olive oil (0g carbohydrates)
* 1/2 tsp paprika (0g carbohydrates)
* Salt and pepper to taste (0g carbohydrates)

Method

1. Preheat the oven to 400°F (200°C).

2. Toss the cooked chickpeas with olive oil, paprika, salt, and pepper.

3. Spread the chickpeas on a baking sheet and bake for 20-25 minutes, until crispy.

4. Serve the roasted chickpeas and enjoy.

Total Carbohydrates

14g carbohydrates (chickpeas, olive oil)

Recipe 10: Vegan Smoothie Bowl

Ingredients and Carb Counts

* 1 cup frozen mixed berries (21g carbohydrates)
* 1/2 cup unsweetened almond milk (0g carbohydrates)
* 1/4 cup cooked quinoa (6g carbohydrates)
* 1 tbsp chia seeds (3g carbohydrates)
* 1 tbsp chopped nuts (1g carbohydrates)

Method

1. In a blender, combine the frozen mixed berries and almond milk.
2. Blend until smooth.
3. Pour the smoothie into a bowl.
4. Top the smoothie with cooked quinoa, chia seeds, and chopped nuts.
5. Serve the smoothie bowl and enjoy.

Total Carbohydrates

32g carbohydrates (mixed berries, quinoa, chia seeds, nuts)

These vegan recipes can be adjusted and modified based on your individual preferences, dietary needs, and carbohydrate allowance. Remember to track the carbohydrates in each ingredient and the total carbohydrates in the final dish to ensure you stay within your desired carb range. Enjoy experimenting with these vegan recipes and discovering new favourites!